Minimizing Post-op Pain

*A 12 Step Program for
Surgical Teams*

Susan A. Crockett, MD

DEDICATION

This guide is dedicated to minimally invasive surgical
pioneers everywhere,
and the patients we serve.

CONTENTS

Preface   1

1   Prepare for the best   Pg 5
2   Prevent pain before it starts   Pg 7
3   Make smaller incisions   Pg 9
4   Make fewer incisions   Pg 11
5   Minimize trauma to the peritoneum   Pg 13
6   Minimize incisional stress and drama   Pg 15
7   Decrease air pressure   Pg 17
8   Prevent adhesions   Pg 19
9   Prevent inflammation   Pg 21
10 Address ALL pathology   Pg 23
11 Constipation is the enemy   Pg 25
12 Train your staff to new expectations   Pg 27

PREFACE

Why not prevent pain at every point possible?

Our team has a pretty fantastic job.

Every week we get to meet together in the OR with the chance to help patients increase their quality of life. In our OR, we say that every case is like Christmas, because although we can do all our history & physical taking, imaging and workup, we never really know what we're getting into until we open it up. That is where the joy and the art of surgery take over. A creative process unlike any other, where our surgical team goes into action to maximize results and minimize our impact on the patient.

The goal is painless, scarless, bloodless surgery.

In this guide, our surgical team is proud to share with you our multimodal pain prevention protocol, based on our experiential knowledge gained from almost 500 robotic cases. Many of our ideas are similar to those developed and shared by ERAS (Enhanced Recovery After Surgery) Society. http://www.erassociety.org/

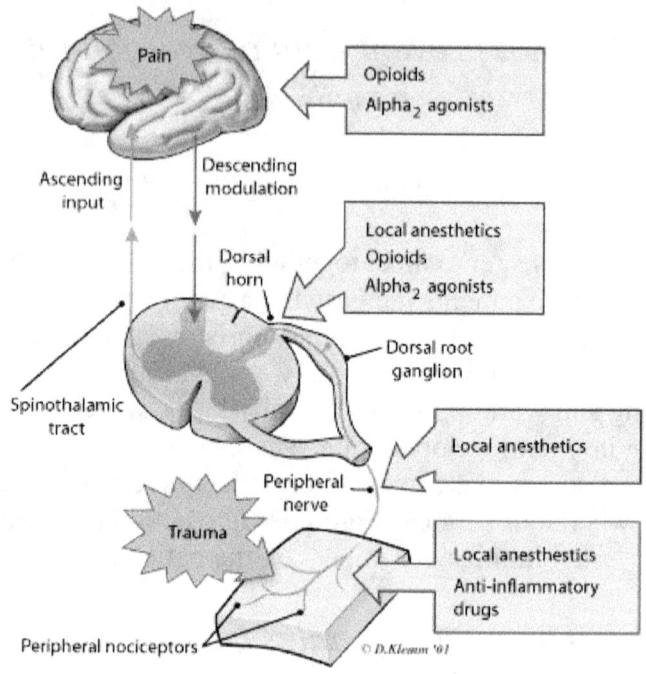

Pain

Opioids
Alpha$_2$ agonists

Ascending input

Descending modulation

Local anesthetics
Opioids
Alpha$_2$ agonists

Dorsal horn

Dorsal root ganglion

Spinothalamic tract

Local anesthetics

Peripheral nerve

Trauma

Local anesthestics
Anti-inflammatory drugs

Peripheral nociceptors

© D.Klemm '01

from Kehlet H, Dahl JB. The value of "multimodal" or "balanced analgesia" in postoperative pain treatment. AnesthAnalg 1993;77:1049.

In addition to sharing with you our "hard science" methods of approaching the pain pathways show in this figure to the left, we will also be sharing some very practical and powerful psychological tools we use to enhance the postoperative experience for patients (and make you the hero with them!) We are in private practice, so we are completely dependent on patient satisfaction for maintaining a financially stable and successful practice. Reputation is gold.

Although our specialty is minimally invasive benign gyn, it is our hope that you will find useful techniques in this program that will translate to your field of surgery as well.

1
PREPARE FOR THE BEST

Successful surgical outcomes begin in the office with intentional pre-operative counseling.

Call it placebo effect, hypnotic suggestion, peer pressure, the power of suggestion or positive thinking....call it whatever you want.....

but we have found that preparing the patient to *expect* minimal pain and possibly *no* pain after surgery may be one of the most important steps in mitigating the *experience* of elevated postoperative pain.

- Before surgery, with the patient *and their family*, we review the multimodal steps we take to decrease the patient's pain and educate them on the importance of the steps that they participate in (bowel care, scheduled NSAID regimens, early ambulation).
- We also talk to them about what typical patient (peer) usage is for post-op rescue narcotic pain relievers (2-5 Tylenol #3 tablets, total, in the post-op period).
- We teach them not to medicate down to a pain score of 0, but rather to tolerate the level of soreness they would expect after a hard workout, without adding narcotic rescue medication.

"You wouldn't take codeine for the soreness you would feel after doing a hundred sit-ups, would you?"

2
PREVENT PAIN BEFORE IT STARTS

Practice preemptive analgesia with a
long-acting local anesthetic.

By pre-injecting our incisions with local anesthetic, we have the opportunity to stop pain before it starts by down-regulating the nerve fibers (see diagram on page 2). See? Local anesthetics act at three different levels of pain to inhibit afferent nerve input:

- Peripheral nociceptors
- Peripheral nerve
- Nerve root

By varying the type of local anesthetic we use, we can extend pre-emptive analgesia into the post-operative period. Our team has gone through an evolution of trying different local anesthetics, listed from top to bottom below:

- Lidocaine - wears off before the end of surgery
- Bupivacaine - lasts a little longer (2-9 hours) but has cardiovascular risks
- Ropivicaine - 1-3 hours, less cardiovascular risk
- EXPAREL (depafoam bupivacaine) maintains blood concentrations 3-5 days

For robotic cases, we use a dilution of 20cc of EXPAREL in 100cc of injectable saline. Half is used for pre-injection, half for pelvic bath.

3
MAKE SMALLER INCISIONS

Smaller incisions mean less pain, less risk of infection, and less risk of traumatic disruption, especially for obese patients.

Top robotic surgeons in benign gyn shoot for a <5% open laparotomy rate. This includes both their conversion rate and planned open surgeries. Many achieve sustainable 1-2% open rates.

We have found that small incision surgery using robotic technology is especially beneficial for obese patients, affording better access, visualization, and manipulation in the center of a thicker body. Also, the movement of the panus postoperatively as the patient becomes upright is no insignificant stressor to the abdominal wall. Smaller incisions not only hurt less, but they also have a smaller risk of infection and subcutaneous traumatic internal hemorrhage.

Are there times when a large open incision is necessary? Absolutely. But most benign pathology can be safely and quickly removed through small incision surgery.

Our team strives for "no more large incisions."

4
MAKE FEWER INCISIONS

Fewer incisions = less pain (most of the time)

It may seem intuitive that fewer incisions would result in less pain. Our team has seen that be the case for most approaches to intra-abdominal surgeries with the exception of the vaginal approach, the "original incision-less" surgery. Not only does the vaginal approach to pelvic surgery seriously limit the surgeons visibility, and ability to identify critical complicating pathology, but we have also seen considerably more pain from the stress of pulling the ovaries and infundibulopelvic ligaments from the level of the iliac crest to the level of the pelvic floor. Here are some of our favorite "fewer incision" options:

- single site laparoscopic or robotic surgery - single incision usually hidden completely in the umbilicus. All ports for camera, instruments, and assistant go through this single multiport.
- reduced port laparoscopic or robotic surgery - useful for cases that start out as single site, but may require a "one off" laparoscopic port for a robotic tool or assistant port. Helpful for suction, retraction, and passing needles or tissue.
- low impact instrumentation - these latest laparoscopic tools are 2-3mm in diameter, leaving almost no incision. Advances in technology have made them stronger and more versatile than using a full port, as they can be moved from site to site as need during a case. Our favorite is the MiniLap Alligator Grasper (http://www.teleflex.com/en/usa/spotlight/mini-lap/)

5
MINIMIZE TRAUMA TO THE PERITONEUM

Use fine surgical techniques to minimize disruption to the peritoneal surface.

When I was in residency, I came across a book called "The Art of Surgical Technique," by Milton T. Edgerton. Now, some 20+ years later, I still carry with me his lessons about gentle handling of tissue, choice of instruments, needles, and sutures, and fine surgical techniques. Laparoscopy, and now robotic surgery, have brought additional levels of finesse to the operative field for preventing tissue damage. I tell my patients sometimes that for me, the difference between operating laparoscopically vs. robotically, is the difference between an artist drawing with a box of 8 crayons vs. painting with oils. As our team has progressed from open, through laparoscopic, to roboitc surgery, we have adopted the following rules for handling tissue:

- leave a low surgical footprint - touch and disrupt as little as possible. The deep trendelenburg positioning we use in robotic pelvic surgery minimizes the need to handle bowel, reducing pain, scarring, and ileus.
- don't leave hardware behind - this includes bands, clips, staples, etc...
- use gentle surgical technique - handle the tissue with respect and minimize charring
- leave a low surgical footprint - touch and disrupt as little as possible. The deep trendelenburg positioning we use in robotic pelvic surgery

Always aspire to do your best.

6
MINIMIZE INCISIONAL STRESS & DRAMA

The bigger the bandage, the bigger the pain.

Have you ever noticed the difference in patient response to their incisions based on the dressings? Often, the bigger and thicker the dressing, the more the patient assumes a larger incision and more therefore more dramatic pain. One psychological way of addressing this is by using band aids instead of bandages. Even better, no bandage. We close with subcuticular sutures and Dermabond. In addition to seeming less dramatic to the patient, they can shower immediately without messing with gunky gluey bandages and the sterile field is maintained for a few days after the surgery.

Additionally, because they are positioned on a fulcrum, robotic trocars are less likely to cause stress on the incisions than their laparoscopic counterparts.

Less stress = less pain.

"The pain of the mind is worse than the pain of the body."

Pubilius Syrus (1st Century BC-?)Roman writer and poet

7
DECREASE AIR PRESSURE

*Now that we've developed ways to decrease incisional and
bowel pain, shoulder pain from
intra-abdominal gas pressure during surgery is our #1
postop pain complaint.*

After laparoscopic surgery, referred pain from the phrenic
nerve can sometimes cause considerable shoulder pain, and
we have found this to be one of the most challenging
postoperative problems to address. Our team has
experimented with a few ways to successfully deal with
postoperative shoulder pain.

- eliminate as much excess CO_2 from the abdominal
  cavity by opening the trocars and squeezing as
  much air out as possible
- give 5 positive pressure ventilations by anesthesia at
  the end of the case
- use lower intraoperative gas pressures by using a
  balloon trocar as a retractor for the anterior
  abdominal wall
- use a low pressure insufflation system such as
  SurgiQuest's AirSeal device (LOVE this device for
  so many other features as well!)

8
PREVENT ADHESIONS

Adhesions from prior surgery are a significant cause of chronic pain, bowel obstruction, and long term disability.

There is no perfect adhesion barrier, but any of the ones listed below are better than nothing in most cases. By not using adhesion barriers, you are setting your patient up for risk of chronic pain and future surgical issues. There is some indication that newer modalities, such as amniotic cells or membranes, may actually work to decrease reformation of lysed adhesions by preventing the scarring cascade at the cellular level through germ cell mechanisms.

- use fine surgical technique to decrease tissue damage (see #5)
- use adhesion prevention products - Sprafilm, Surgiwrap, Adept, Interceed, Evicel, Goretex
- Next generation, currently in study - Regenerative Tissue Grafts - amniotic membrane grafts. Widely used in prostatectomy and spine surgery. Some promise for bowel and gyn surgery adhesion prevention
- Get bowel moving quickly (see #11)

A chance to cut is a chance to cure, unless more damage is caused than fixed!

9
PREVENT INFLAMMATION

Inflammation is the enemy of healing and health.

So much that we've already discussed has to do with decreasing inflammation. However, we think inflammation deserves it's own mention, as it is a key (maybe THE key) to preventing postoperative pain. As illustrated by the diagram on the left (from http://www.arthritis.co.za/arachid.html), we can decrease the inflammatory response first by limiting the stimulus (see #2-9) and secondarily by blocking the cascade or end products at the tissue level.

Our team uses IM ketorolac as a prostaglandin inhibitor, injected at the end of almost every case, except in those cases where it is contraindicated, in which case IV acetaminophen is given instead. We follow this by a scheduled regimen of 600mg of ibuprofen every 6 hours for 3-5 days following surgery. In our experience we have found that this not only decreases the inflammatory pain response, but it also decreases the need for narcotics postoperatively when used in combination with EXPAREL local anesthetic.

***Our team also recommends a whole foods vegetable based diet postoperatively,
high in fresh fruits & green vegetables,
low in inflammatory additives.***

10
ADDRESS ALL PATHOLOGY

Address all possible pathology at the time of surgery.
The operative word here is "ALL."

I know that this might sound basic, but it is important, and I'm not mentioning anything here that our team hasn't experienced in real life practice. First, it is impossible to treat ALL sources of pain if you don't look or you can't see it.

"There are none so blind as those who will not see."
Proverb

This our team's greatest argument against the vaginal approach to intra-abdominal pelvic surgery. Additionally, robotic surgery prepares a surgeon to very quickly and easily take care of most minor causes of pain such as adhesions, leftover hardware (clips, bands, staples, etc....) or additional pathologic conditions not identified prior to surgery, such as endometriosis or infection, and thus should be consider the gold standard for pelvic pain cases.

Finally, we realize that not all sources of pain can be known ahead of time, and sometimes they require a second surgery or coordination with a different surgical team. That's why we always say...

Surgery is like Christmas!
You never know what you're going to find once you open.

11
CONSTIPATION IS THE ENEMY

Empty the bowel prior to surgery and keep it moving afterwards.

For pelvic surgery in general, and for robotic surgery in particular, a full colon is the enemy. Not only does it take up precious space which represents our safety margin for the operative field, but it poses a physical threat to the maintenance of postoperative pain control. Imagine rocks scraping on the inside of an incision site. Add on top of that, the pain and risk caused by straining, and we have a full fledged enemy.

We recommend bowel prep prior to surgery, not squeeky clean, but emptied, and stool softeners after surgery to maintain 2-3 soft bowel movements a day. Since patients vary greatly in their response to bowel stimulants, our team does not have a standard recommendation. We ask the patient to ambulate early, and choose whatever works for them. Maybe fiber or Colase, might need Miralax or Dulcolax. The toughest cases sip on Magnesium Citrate to keep things moving until they normalize. Also, we maximize non-narcotic pain control postop in order to decrease narcotic induced constipation.

"Don't mess with Mr. Stinky!"

12
TRAIN YOUR STAFF FOR NEW EXPECTATIONS

Educate your postoperative team to give less narcotic medication in the postop period.

Your post-op nurses will start to see the differences themselves (and will love you for making their job easier) without you even telling them, but in general, you should train your patients, family, and postoperative nurses to expect lower levels of pain, and less use of narcotics when implementing the multimodal pain control steps detailed in this program. Make sure to set their expectations for less pain and less need for narcotic use. Explain to them the things your team is doing change patients' postoperative experiences as you become an innovator in minimally invasive surgery and invite them to become part of the less-narcotic-use medical community.

Teach them to resist the urge to give narcotics TO PREVENT more severe pain, but to give them only FOR TREATMENT of severe pain.

We typically write prescriptions for ibuprofen and tylenol #3, using the tylenol #3 only as a breakthrough pain medicine. Our office staff is trained for the same instructions and expectations.

How low can you go?
How much pain can you help your patients NOT experience?

MINIMIZING POSTOP PAIN
A 12 Step Program for Surgical Teams

CHEAT SHEET

1. Prepare for the best
2. Prevent pain before it starts
3. Make smaller incisions
4. Make fewer incisions
5. Minimize trauma to the peritoneum
6. Minimize incisional stress & drama
7. Decrease air pressure
8. Prevent adhesions
9. Prevent inflammation
10. Address ALL pathology
11. Constipation is the enemy
12. Train your staff to new expectations

ABOUT BOTDOCS

If you liked this guide, then you'll love

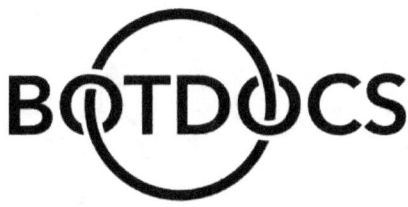

Come join our team as we prepare to launch the first online medical education platform of its kind, dedicated to sharing our collective knowledge of robotic surgical products, practices, & techniques.

We are bringing medical education up to the speed of NOW, incorporating technological advancements to reconnect surgeons of all levels in a personal & real time way.

We look forward to meeting you at BotDocs.com!

www.ingramcontent.com/pod-product-compliance
Lightning Source LLC
Chambersburg PA
CBHW071831200526
45169CB00018B/1361